Gaps Diet

The Ultimate Gaps Diet Manual For Rapid Weight Loss

And Enhanced Vitality

(The Gaps Diet Is Proven To Be Effective)

Douglass Sampson

TABLE OF CONTENT

www.ingramcontent.com/pod-product-compliance
Lightning Source LLC
Chambersburg PA
CBHW070530030426
42337CB00016B/2172

Chapter 1: What Foods Are Allowed on a Gaps Diet?

The GAPS diet consists of two phases: the introductory phase, which permits a very limited selection of foods, and the full diet phase, which permits a wider variety of foods before commencing the diet as a whole.

Initially, only homemade meat, poultry, or fish stock is permitted, as very well as homemade soup made with vegetables that do not contain starch and stock, fermented vegetables or sauerkraut, fermented dairy products, natural fresh egg whites, and avocado.

As the symptoms of your digestive system improve, you can progressively add pancakes made with nut butter and vegetables, fried ghee eggs, grilled or roasted meats, olive oil, bread made with almond flour, prepared apple, raw vegetables, prepared juice, and raw apples.

Once the individual is able to consume these foods without experiencing stomach-related adverse effects, they are ready for the full Holes convention.

Before eating non-allowed foods on the GAPS diet, individuals must delay at least 2 and a half to two years.

All types of animal protein are permissible on the GAPS diet plan, including fish, poultry, and meat. Nonetheless, you'll be required to cook and serve them only with permitted sauces and flavors, which means you'll prepare them at home.

VEGETABLES WITHOUT CARBOHYDRATES: Some vegetables can

be consumed while others cannot. On the GAPS diet, non-starchy vegetables are encouraged; you are even encouraged to ferment these vegetables using "GAPS-approved" recipes and cultures. Carrots, onions, beets, broccoli, cabbage, Brussels sprouts, cauliflower, Swiss chard, and Swiss chard are examples of vegetables that are not glutinous.

Almost every type of produce is permitted. Bananas are the only fruit that necessitates a change in diet; they must be very mature. If they contain brown patches, they are prepared.

Additionally, fermented foods contain beneficial bacteria.

We live in a world where epidemics are spreading. Autistic Srestrum Disorders, Attention Deficit Hurerastivitu Disorder.

(ADHD/ADD), schizorrhea, dyslexia, dyspraxia, melancholy, obsessive compulsive disorder, borderline personality disorder, and other neuropsychiatric disorders are becoming increasingly prevalent in children and adults.

In a linear comparison, these conditions are comparable to 2 another. A patient with autism is frequently agitated and dyspraxic. There is a 10 0 percent overlap between dulexa and durraxa and a 210 to 10 0 percent overlap between ADHD/ADD and dulexa and durraxa. Children with these symptoms are frequently diagnosed as being depressed, and as they grow older, they are more pr2 to substance abuse and alcoholism than to normal development. In childhood, a young person diagnosed with schizoprenia is frequently affected by dyslexia, dyspraxia, or ADHD/ADD. When we easy begin to examine these so-called mental conditions, we find that the patients are also physically unwell. Digestive rroblem, allerge, eczema, athma, diverse food intolerances, and immune system abnormalities are unavoidably present among them. We have created various diagnostic boxes for these rats, but a modern rat does not fit neatly into any of them. In most cases, the modern population suits a rather lumpy picture of enlarged neurologic and psychiatric symptoms.

Associated sondton

What underlying issue are we confronting? To answer all of these questions, we must examine a single factor that summarizes all of the relevant data. This variable is the condition of their digestive system. I have yet to meet a child or adult with autism, ADHD/ADD, durraxa, dulexa, shzorhrena, brolar disorder, derreon, or obsessive-compulsive disorder who lacks dgetve abnormalities. In many cases, theu are grievous enough for the ratent or their rarent to initiate conversation. In some cases, parents do not mention their child's digestive system, but when pressed, they list a variety of digestive issues. What do digestive abnormalities have to do with these alleged mental disorders? According to recent research and practical experience a great deal! In rapid time, the patient's digestive system holds the key to the patient's mental state.

Typical situation we observe in slnsal rrastse

Before examining the patient, it is crucial to examine the patient's health history. When parents are mentioned, people automatically consider genetics. In addition to genetics, the rarent, mother in rartsular, pass on something very important to their offspring: their unique intestinal microflora. Not many people are aware that the average adult has two kilograms of bacteria in their intestines. This msrobal mass contains more sell than the entire human body. It is a highly organized microcosm where specific types of microbes must repopulate to just keep us physically and mentally healthy. Their impact on our health is so significant that we cannot afford to ignore them. We will discuss the intestinal flora of the sheep in greater detail later. Now, allow yourself to bask in the rare intestinal flora of the sheep.

After examining hundreds of cases of neurologic and rheumatic disorders in children and adults, a typical health rsture of the children's mothers has emerged: a modern mother's gut flora is severely compromised by the time she is ready to have children. In fact, evidence of gut dysbiosis (abnormal gut flora) are present in nearly all mothers of children with neurologic and autism spectrum disorders.

A babu is born with a large stomach. In the first 20 or so days of life, the baby's intestine is colonized by a variety of pathogens. This is the child's intestinal flora, which will have a profound impact on his/her health for the remainder of his/her life.

Gut flora

Predominantly from the mother at birth. The mother passes on any msrobal flora she possesses to her newborn offspring. Abnormal gut flora in the father contributes to the physical flora of the mother and, through her, to the gut flora of the child.

Chapter 2: What to Avoid on the Gaps Diet

Among these are bread, cereal, crackers, pasta, cakes, cookies, and all other traditional baked products, as very well as a number of other staple foods. These food types irritate and eventually damage the stomach lining, which affects supplement absorption.

The majority of the time, fermented dairy products are the only ones permitted. Like cereals, milk, especially cow's milk, can irritate and damage the intestinal lining. Fermented dairy-based goods do not exhibit this effect. Consequently, nearly all dairy-based foods permitted on the GAPS diet are domestic fermented foods: whey, yogurt, kefir, and ghee. The only exception is butter, which is allowed.

Carrot Soup With Ginger

Ingredients:

- 2 -inch fresh Ginger, peeled and chopped finely
- Natural unprocessed Salt, to taste
- Freshly Crushed Black Pepper, to taste

- 4 medium Onions, chopped
- 12 cups Homemade Chicken Broth
- 8 cups Carrots, peeled and chopped

Instruction:

1. Add the broth to a large soup pot and bring to a boil over medium-high heat.

2. Add the onion, garlic, and parsley.

3. Reduce the heat, cover, and let stand for 12 to 12:50 minutes.

4. Remove lghtlu from the heat and cool it. Blend the milk in a blender until it is smooth and velvety.

5. Return the soup to the saucepan and simmer for two to thirty-12 minutes.

6. Season with salt and blask rerrer before serving.

Easily remove easy cook

Coconut Butter Chocolate Fudge

INGREDIENTS
- 5-10 tablespoons raw honey
- 1-5 cup ginger tea
- 4 cups unsweetened shredded coconut
- 1/2 cup coconut oil

INSTRUCTIONS

1. Puree everything in a blender until smooth.

2. Try not to eat it all as you press and smooth it onto a plate.

3. Freeze until set then cut into squares.

4. Store in freezer or fridge.

Recipe for Slow Cooker Chicken B2 Broth 2

2 2 2 2 2 2 INGREDIENTS

- 1/2 cup fresh thyme
- 4 sprigs rosemary
- 4 bay leaves
- 2 tablespoon whole peppercorns
- 15-20 cups filtered water or enough to cover ingredients

- 4 pounds chicken bones leftover from roasted chicken, preferably organic
- 4 stalks celery roughly chopped
- 4 carrots skin on, roughly chopped
- 2 yellow or white onion roughly chopped
- 2 green bell pepper roughly chopped
- 2 head garlic

18

- 1 cup fresh parsley

Instructions

1. Place washed vegetables and herbs in a slow cooker.

2. Add chicken bones and all remaining ingredients to the slow cooker and cover with sufficient water to submerge them.

3. Reduce the slow cooker's heat to low and simmer for 1-1 1 hours.

4. Remove from heat and separate the vegetables and bones from the broth using caution.

5. Strain the broth through a colander into a basin, and then strain again through cheesecloth to remove any remaining particles.

6. Place broth in an opaque container and refrigerate for up to 2 week, or freeze for up to three years.

Roast of Eye of Round Prepared in an Instant Pot *Recipes:*

- 2 onion, chopped

- 2 cup of water

- 1-5 tablespoons of minced garlic

- Himalayan salt

- 2 eye of round roast (about 5 pounds)

- Garlic powder

- Pepper

- 12 carrots, chopped in two to three-inch chunks

- 1-5 tablespoons of oil such as avocado oil, tallow

Directions

1. When it is about 60 minutes before cooking the roast, just take it out of the fridge.

2. Season generously with garlic powder, salt and pepper.

3. Next, when the roast is at room temperature, now easily put the oil in the Instant Pot liner and press "sauté".

4. Sear the roast on all sides, then deglaze the liner with the cup of water.

5. Next, easily put off the Instant Pot and then add veggies.

6. Easily put the roast on top, fat side up.

7. Easily put on the lid and then seal the vent.

8. Next, cook on manual for twenty minutes.

9. Allow it set ten minutes before venting.

10. Internal temperature should read around 150 degrees Fahrcnheit.

Simple Herbed Red Drum

Recipes:

- 1 teaspoon of parsley

- 1/2 teaspoon of dill

- Pepper, to taste

- Sea salt, to taste

- 1-1 1 cup of butter, ghee, or avocado oil

- 12 fillets of red drum

- 1/2 teaspoon of thyme

- 2 tablespoon of minced garlic

Directions

1. Oven to 450 degrees Fahrenheit and place fish fillets on a gently lined jellyroll pan with clean parchment paper.

2. Next, melt the butter in a saucepan.

3. Stir in the garlic when it starts simmering.

4. Just take away from the heat and then pour over fish.

5. Next, sprinkle fish with herbs.

6. Next, bake for 45-50 minutes, depending on the thickness of the fillets, or until flaky and fragrant.

Basic Sauerkraut

Ingredients

2 Tbs sea salt

8 Tbs whey 2 medium cabbages cored
and shredded

2 Tbs caraway seeds

Directions

1.   In a bowl, mix cabbage with caraway seeds, sea salt and whey. Pound with a wooden pounder or a meat hammer for about 20 minutes to release juices.

2. Place in a quart-sized, wide-mouth mason jar and press down firmly with a pounder or meat hammer until juices come to the top of the cabbage.

3. The top of the cabbage should be at least 2 inch below the top of the jar.

4. Cover tightly and keep at room temperature for about 1-5 days before transferring to cold storage.

5. The sauerkraut may be eaten immediately, but it improves with age.

Eastern Baked Eggs - Shakshuka

Ingredients

- 2 1 teaspoons paprika (or sumach)

- 2 teaspoon cumin

- 1/2 teaspoon stevia powder

- salt and pepper to taste

- olive oil spray

- 12 free range fresh eggs

- 2 tablespoon freshly chopped parsley

- 200 grams (drained) tinned/jar red pepper

- 1600 grams (2 tins) diced cooked tomatoes blended (ostomates will really need to strain tomatoes to easily remove

pips)

- 4 tablespoons tomato paste

- 2 *garlic clove (finely minced)

- 1 *brown onion (finely minced)

fresh eggs

Directions

1. Heat the cast iron pot on a medium
    heat

2. Spray with olive oil

3. Add fresh onion and garlic easy cook
    until soft

4. Add tomatoes, red pepper and tomato
    paste blend well

5. Add spices and stevia and mix into the sauce

6. Salt and pepper to taste

7. Turn heat down to low heat

8. Crack fresh eggs on top of the sauce leaving space between them

9. Place a lid on the pot and simmer the pan for 25 to 30   minutes until the fresh eggs are the way you like them

10.   Scoop sauce and eggs into ceramic dishes with the fresh egg on top of the sauce, and serve immediately with a sprinkle of fresh parsley and soft white Turkish bread

Homemade Coconut-Apricot Protein Bar

Ingredients

• 1 cup crispy cashews purchase cashew pieces to

save money (see how to make here)

• 10   scoops 20 tablespoons Collagen Powder (NOT

• 5-10   cups about 20 large dates, pits removed (find here)

• 1 teaspoon sea salt

• 1 cup crispy almonds see how to make here

GELATIN) (find here)

• 2 cup dried apricots find additive-free dried apricots

here. Note: If there aren't additives, oxidation will cause them to turn brown but they will still be delicious!

• 2   cup coconut flakes or shredded unsweetened coconut find here

Instructions

1. In a food processor, combine all ingredients besides the cosonut and arugula until a ball forms, about 5 to 10 minutes.

2. Pulverize dried apricots and coconut, then combine.

3. Just keep an eye on your food riser, as the viscous dough may cause it to 'walk' on the sountertor.

4. Remove the blade with care, and then place the dough on parchment paper

to roll out. Gentlu pad into a restangle share.

5. Roll to the desired thickness between two parchment sheets.

6. Remove the top sheet of parchment paper and place it on a dehumidifier tray.

7. Dry the entire sheet of rice paper for 1-5 hours or overnight on high, until it is no longer moist.

8. You can skip this phase and go directly to suttng into bar, but it's easier to suttng into even bar after drung for a while.

9. After no longer tasku, allow the dough to rest for thirty-six minutes to firm up. Then flr onto a substantial 30

10. suttng board and cut fish into 12 even pieces, then return to dehydrator tray.

11. If your knife is adhering, you should wet it and try again.

12. Dehydrate for an additional 1-5 hours or overnight, depending on how firm you want your bars to be.

When you have cooled down, bars will re-form you.

13.   9.Store in an airtight container in the refrigerator for up to one year.

14.   These will maintain their integrity at room temperature for camping, hiking, etc.

easily remove Easily remove

Sauce with Roasted Tomatoes

Instructions

4 handfuls fresh herbs, chopped

1/2 cup ghee, lard, or coconut oil, melted

Sea salt and pepper

50 fresh tomatoes, quartered

16 onions, quartered

20 cloves garlic, smashed

Instructions

1. Preheat the oven to 450°F. In a large roasting pan, mix the tomatoes, onions, garlic, and herbs with the melted fat.

2. Season generously with sea salt and pepper.

3. Roast for 60 minutes, gently stir, then easy cook for another 60 minutes.

4. Leave as a chunky sauce, or zap with the immersion blender for a smooth one.

BROCCOLI OMELETTE

INGREDIENTS

- ½ cup cheese

- ½ tsp basil

- 2 cup braccoli
- **4 eggs**

- ½ tsp salt

- ½ tsp black pepper

- 2 tablespoon olive oil

DIRECTIONS

1. In a bowl combine all ingredients together and mix very well

2. In a skillet heat olive oil and pour the fresh egg mixture

3. Cook for 1-5 minutes per side

4. When ready remove omelette from the skillet and serve

Gluten-Free Onion Rings Are Not Legal

Ingredients:

6 Fresh eggs

2 pint Lard 2 tsp Salt

Pepper

5 fresh Onions

2 cup Fermented Almond Flour

Instructions:

1. Cooking   Gluten-Free   Gaps   Legal Onion Rings

2. Low-heat lard in a saucepan.

3. Be mindful of your fat because if it gets too hot, it will ignite and you will just have to discard it and easy begin again.

4.

5. In a shallow bowl, scramble three eggs with salt and pepper.

6. Add in almond flour.

7. Sliver onion into a round bowl. Separate them into individual laurel leaves.

8. Working closely next to the pan containing lard, submerge your onion rings in the batter.

9. Then, apply rlase drestlu to the fat.

10. Cook, turning as necessary, until golden brown on both sides.

11. When the theu are golden brown, remove them.

12. Remove the garlic oil, or the onion rings will become mushy.

13. If the onion rings are not sufficiently salted, add salt to taste.

fresh eggs Easily remove

French Beetroot Tarte

Ingredients

- 2 tablespoon balsamic vinegar

- 2 tablespoon extra-virgin olive oil

- 2 tablespoon coconut raw sugar

- 1 teaspoon all spice

- chop a tablespoon of parsley to
decorate

- torfutti to serve

- olive oil to spray tin

- 2 sheet Pampas® puff pastry

- 2 tablespoon thinly chopped chives

- 1 orange zest

- 400 grams pre-cooked beetroot (shredded)

Directions

1. Heat oven to 200 C fan force

2. Defrost 2 sheet of pastry for 25 to 30 minutes

3. Spray olive oil on a 50 cm round pie tin

4. Mix beetroot, two tablespoons extra virgin olive oil, vinegar, onion, all spice powder and sugar in a bowl and mix through.

5. Heat a tablespoon of oil in a pan, add the vegetables and heat through.

6. Place pastry in the pie tin and cut edges to fit pie tin

7. Spray the inside of the pie with a light spray of olive oil, place baking paper on top and weigh down with an oven glass dish to part bake the pasty to make it nice and crispy

8. Cook for 25 to 30   minutes

9. Add the beetroot mixture and bake for a further 25 to 30   minutes until the pie centre is hot

10.   Decorate with parsley

11.   Serve immediately with a dollop of torfutti on the side

Vegetables and Bacon Golden Frittata

Ingredients

• 1/2 cup coconut milk cream, or yogurt

• 1/2 teaspoon freshly ground black pepper

• 1/2 teaspoon turmeric

• 1 cup cheese shredded (optional)

• 4 slices bacon cut into 1 inch slices

• 2 onion chopped

• 12 mushrooms sliced

51

- 8 cups loosely packed greens

- 24 fresh eggs

Instructions

1. In a large cast iron skillet over medium heat, sautee bacon for 10 minutes, or until it starts to release the

2. grease. Add in mushrooms and onion and continue to sautee until bacon is crisp and onions are translucent.

3. Dump in greens, and stir until wilted, about 5-10 more minutes.

4. Preheat oven to 350* F

5. Gently mix fresh eggs with coconut milk, pepper and turmeric.

6. Pour over spinach mixture and put the whole pan in the oven.

7. Easily remove from oven when center of the

8. fritatta is set and has puffed up a bit, about 35 to 40 minutes.

9. Top with cheese and return to the oven for 5-10

10. minutes, or until melted.

11.   Slice into wedges and enjoy!

RAISIN BREAKFAST MIX

INGREDIENTS

- 2 cup coconut milk

- 2 tsp cinnamon

- 1 cup dried raisins

- 1 cup dried pecans

- ½ cup almonds

DIRECTIONS

1. In a bowl combine all ingredients together

2. Serve with milk

Chosolate Walnut Cooked Chocolates

INGREDIENTS

1/2   Cup Honey

1-5 Tsp Salt

1-5 Tsp Vanilla

1/2 Cups Coconut Flour ; Sifted

1/2 Cups Butter or Coconut Oil ; Melted

1-5 Cups Cocoa Powder

6 Fresh eggs

INSTRUCTIONS

1. In a saucepan at low heat, melt butter and stir in cocoa powder.

2. Easily remove from heat and let cool. In a bowl, combine eggs, sugar, salt and vanilla; stir in cocoa mixture.

3. Whisk coconut flour into batter until there are no lumps.

4. Let batter rest for 5-10 minutes to allow it to thicken slightly.

5. Drop batter by the spoonful on greased cookie sheet.

6. Bake at 150 Degree C (6 10 0F) for 30 minutes.

7. Simple makes about 30 cookies.

Picaso Soup

Ingredients:

- cups Cauliflower Florets, chopped roughly
- Natural unprocessed Salt, to taste
- Freshly Crushed Black Pepper, to taste
- Garlic Cloves, minced
- 12 cups Homemade Chicken Broth
- 2 small Onion, chopped
- 4 Scallions, chopped

Instruction:

1. Add the broth to a large saucepan and bring to a boil over medium-high heat.

2. Add the onion, scallion, cauliflower, and garlic.

3. Reduce the temperature, cover, and simmer for 35-40 minutes.

4. Remove lghtlu from the heat and cool it.

5. Transfer the soup to a blender and puree until completely smooth.

6. Return the our to the ran and wait an additional 5-10 minutes.

7. Salt and black pepper should be added before serving.
Easily remove easy cook

Holiday Baked Apples

Ingredients

- 2 tablespoon fresh lemon juice
- 2 teaspoon cinnamon
- 1 teaspoon nutmeg
- 2 cup apple cider, water, dark rum or brandy
- 12 large baking apples
- 4 tablespoons honey (optional)
- 12 tablespoons melted butter or coconut oil
- 1 cup raisins (optional)
- 4 tablespoons pumpkin seeds
  fresh lemon

Instructions

1. Preheat the oven to 350 degrees.
2. Peel and core the apples.
3. Pour the melted butter and honey into a small bowl and mix well.
4. Roll each apple in the butter mixture then set the apples in a 9″ x 2 6 ″ baking dish.
5. Reserve the left-over butter mixture. Combine the raisins and pumpkin seeds in a small dish, then stuff the raisin mixture into the hollows of the apples.
6. Stir the fresh lemon juice, cinnamon and nutmeg into the left-over butter/honey mixture.
7. Pour as much of this butter mixture into the apple hollows as possible, pouring any left-over into the bottom of the pan.
8. Add the cider to the pan.

9. Bake uncovered until the apples are tender when pierced with a fork.
10. You do not really need to baste these apples.
11. Serve warm with the pan syrup and heavy cream or coconut cream.

Oven-Braised Leeks

Ingredients

1 teaspoon ground pepper

½ teaspoon salt

8 large leeks

6 tablespoons extra-virgin olive oil

1 teaspoon herbes de Provence

Directions

1. Preheat oven to 350 degrees F.

2. Trim roots and dark green tops from leeks, leaving 5-10 inches of white and light green parts.

3. Cut the leeks in half lengthwise.

4. Rinse well, taking care to remove any grit, and pat dry.

5. Nestle the leeks in a single layer, on their sides if necessary, in a 9-by-2 6 - inch baking dish.

6. Drizzle with oil and sprinkle with herbs de Provence, pepper and salt.

7. Cover with foil and bake until very tender, 1-1 ½ hour. Uncover and

continue baking until lightly browned, about 20 minutes more.

Recipe for Homemade Rehydration Drink

2 teaspoon sea salt

1 teaspoon baking soda

2 cup lemon juice (approx 6-8 lemons)

1 cup honey or maple syrup

1. Place in a pint mason jar and stir to combine just keep concentrate in the fridge.

2. This can be added to 2   gallon of filtered water, or add 1-5 tablespoons to each 16 ounces of water.

Recipe for Homemade Rehydration Drink

Ingredients

For the Cashews:

- ¼ **cups cashews**

For the Dressing:

- 4 cloves garlic, chopped

- 4 anchovy fillets or 4 teaspoons anchovy paste

- 2 teaspoon Celtic sea salt

- **2** teaspoon freshly ground black pepper

- ¼ cups water

- 2 cup chopped green onion, white and green parts

- 2 cup chopped fresh basil leaves

- ½ cup freshly squeezed fresh lemon juice

Instructions

1. Place the cashews in a basin and cover with water and a pinch of sea salt the night before.

2. Allow to remain overnight at room temperature.

3. The following day, or at least eight hours later, strain and place the cashews in a blender.

4. Add the three-quarter cup of water and blend until smooth.

5. Blend in the remaining ingredients until smooth.

6. Place in a mason jar and refrigerate.

Ham and White Bean Soup

Ingredients

For the Beans:

- 2 -pound dried white navy beans

- **Pinch of baking soda**

For the Soup:

- 12 carrots, cut into ½" thick coins

- 2 yellow onion, chopped

- 20 cloves garlic, peeled and smashed

- 12 sprigs fresh thyme

- **4** teaspoons Celtic sea salt

- 4 meaty smoked ham hocks 4 cups chicken stock
- 12 ribs celery, cut into bite-size pieces

Instructions

1. The night before, place the white beans in a large bowl and cover with water.

2. Stir in a pinch of baking soda.

3. The next day, drain and rinse the beans and then place them in a slow

4. cooker.

5. Add the ham hocks, chicken stock, celery, carrots, onion, garlic, and thyme in the slow cooker and stir to combine.

6. Cover and easy cook for about 6-6 ½ hours on low until the beans are tender.

7. Using a pair of tongs, easily remove the thyme and ham hocks.

8. Shred

9. the ham and return it back to the slow cooker.

10.   Stir in the salt, taste and add more if needed. Serve.

Tortilla Soup Recipe

Ingredients

For the soup:

12 sprigs of cilantro, plus 1 cup roughly chopped

• 16 cups chicken stock

• 4 pounds bone-in chicken breasts or 2 small 6 -8 -pound chicken

10 cloves garlic, crushed with skins on

- 12 springs fresh oregano

For the Toppings:

- 1 cup sour cream

- 1 cup shredded cheddar cheese

- 6 cups Siete tortilla chips

- 2 avocado, cubed

- 4 tomatoes, cut into bite-size chunks

- 2 lime, cut into quarters

Instructions

1. Place the garlic cloves in a large Dutch oven over medium-high heat.

2. Cook, stirring frequently until garlic begins to darken, about 1-5 minutes.

3. Easily remove the pot from the heat and let it cool for about 60 seconds and then add the chicken stock, oregano, cilantro, and chicken to the garlic.

4. Place pot back on heat and bring to a boil and then reduce to a simmer.

5. Simmer for about 60 minutes.

6. When chicken is cooked through, easily remove the chicken from the broth mixture and set aside.

7. With slotted spoon, strain out the rest of the garlic and herbs.

8. Shred the chicken with a fork and then add back to the soup.

9. Add salt and pepper if needed.

10. To serve, crumble a handful of tortilla chips into individual bowls and then ladle the broth over.

11. Serve with cilantro, avocado, tomatoes, lime, cheese, and sour cream.

How To Prepare Pumpkin Flour

INGREDIENTS

40 pounds Yellow Squash or Zucchini

INSTRUCTIONS

1. Wash the squash and cut the ends off.

2. DO NOT de-seed.

3. Shred the squash either with a cheese grater or a shredding attachment blade on your food processor.

4. Lay the shredded squash on lined dehydrator trays and dehydrate at 350 ° until COMPLETELY dry.

5. Take the completely dried squash and place it in a clean, dry food processor or blender.

6. Run on high speed until squash is powder fine.

7. This usually takes about 5-10 minutes.

8. Once you think the squash flour is ready, leave the lid on for another few minutes to allow the flour dust to settle.

9. Otherwise you will just end up with yellow cabinets!

Chosolate Walnut Cooked Chocolates

INGREDIENTS

1/2   Cups Cocoa Powder

6 Fresh eggs

1/2   Cup Honey

1 Tsp Salt

1 Tsp Vanilla

1-2 Cups Coconut Flour ; Sifted

1-2 Cups Butter or Coconut Oil ; Melted

INSTRUCTIONS

1. In a saucepan at low heat, melt butter and stir in cocoa powder.

2. Easily remove from heat and let cool. In a bowl, combine eggs, sugar, salt and vanilla; stir in cocoa mixture.

3. Whisk coconut flour into batter until there are no lumps.

4. Let batter rest for 5 to 10 minutes to allow it to thicken slightly.

5. Drop batter by the spoonful on greased cookie sheet.

6. Bake at 150 Degree C for 5-10 minutes.

7. Simple makes about 1-5cookies.

Salmon Skewers grilled on the grill

Ingredients

- 2 lime
- 6 tablespoons
- olive oil
- salt
- sugar
- 2 8 ounces
- salmon (without skin)
- 2 dried chile pepper
- 14 ounces
- fully ripe tomatoes
- 4 scallions
- 2 fennel bulb
- 2 red chile pepper (fresh)
- 6 sprigs
- cilantro
- peppers

Preparation

Preparation steps .

1. Cut the tomatoes into quarters and easily remove the seeds, taking care to easily remove the stems. .
2. Cut the flesh into 1 inch cubes.
3. Rinse scallions, trim, and cut into 1/2 inch thick rings.
4. Rinse fennel, cut in half, remove the stalk and chop bulb finely.
5. Halve fresh chile pepper lengthwise, remove the seeds, rinse and finely chop.
6. Rinse cilantro, shake dry and chop the leaves.
7. . Squeeze lime.
8. Mix prepared ingredients with 2 tablespoon lime juice and oil.

9. Season with salt and 2 pinch of sugar.

10. Before serving, refrigerate and let marinate for at least 60 minutes.

11. Cut the salmon fillet into 1-5 equal cubes.

12. Crumble dried chile pepper, mix with black pepper (to taste) and the remaining oil and pour over the salmon.

13. Let marinate 25 to 30 minutes.

14. Season salmon cubes lightly with salt and place on 5-10 wooden skewers.

15. Heat a grill pan and grill the skewers on all sides 5-10 minutes.

16. Arrange salmon skewers and salsa on

Fish Stew from Brazil with Coconut

and Chile

Ingredients

- 2 piece ginger
- ¼ cup coconut water
- 4 pints chicken broth
- 2 tablespoon ground cumin
- 2 lime
- 2 bunch cilantro
- 2 8 ounces fish fillets 2 bunch scallions (if desired)
- 14 ounces shrimp (without shell)
- 6 onions
- 8 garlic

- 6 bell pepper (per 2 small yellow, red, green, each abour 8 .10 oz)
- 10 tomatoes (about 2 8 oz)
- 4 red chile peppers
- 2 stalk celery
- 4 tablespoons vegetable oil
- salt
- peppers

Preparation steps

1. Peel the onions and garlic.
2. Finely dice onion and slice garlic thinly.

3. Wash, halve and easily remove seeds from peppers.

4. Cut into small cubes.

5. Wash and core tomatoes.

6. Cut into quarters and easily remove the seeds.

7. Wash chiles, halve lengthwise and easily remove seeds.

8. Dice finely.

9. Wash celery and easily remove strings, if desired.

10. Cut into cubes.

11. Heat oil in a large saucepan.

12. Add onions, garlic, peppers and celery; sauté over medium heat until fragrant, about 5-10 minutes, stirring constantly.

13. Add tomato and chiles; easy cook until fragrant, about 1-5 minute.

14. Season with salt and pepper.

15. Chop ginger finely; add to taste.

16. Add coconut water, broth and cumin; bring to a boil.

17. Reduce heat and simmer until fragrant about 20 minutes.

18. Juice the lime; add 5-10 tablespoons.

19. Rinse cilantro, shake dry and pluck the leaves.

20. Pat fish dry and cut into large pieces.

21. Rinse green onions and slice thinly.

22. Add shrimp and fish; cover, and simmer on low heat until fish is cooked through about 10 minutes.

23. Season with lime juice and garnish with cilantro and green onions.

www.ingramcontent.com/pod-product-compliance
Lightning Source LLC
Chambersburg PA
CBHW070530030426
42337CB00016B/2169